BASIC DIABETES AID AND FORMULA

Diabetes solutions, dieting and management (do's and don'ts)

Marvin bryan

Table of contents

CHAPTER 1
EVERYTHING YOU NEED TO KNOW ABOUT DIABETES

DIABETES TYPES

Diabetes mellitus, often known as diabetes, is a metabolic condition that produces excessive blood sugar. The hormone insulin transports sugar from the blood into your cells to be stored or utilized for energy. With diabetes, your body either doesn't generate enough insulin or can't efficiently utilize the insulin it does make.

Untreated high blood sugar from diabetes may harm your nerves, eyes, kidneys, and other organs.

There are a few distinct forms of diabetes:

TYPE 1 diabetes is an autoimmune illness. The immune system assaults and kills cells in the pancreas, where insulin is generated. It's unknown what triggers this assault.

About 10 percent of patients with diabetes have these types.

TYPE 2 diabetes happens when your body gets resistant to insulin, and sugar builds up in your blood.

PREDIABETES DIABETES: Prediabetes happens when your blood sugar is higher than usual, but it's not high enough for a diagnosis of type 2 diabetes.

GESTATIONAL DIABETES: this type is elevated blood sugar during pregnancy. Insulin-blocking substances generated by the placenta induce this type of diabetes.

An uncommon illness termed diabetes insipidus is not connected to diabetes mellitus, although it has a similar name. It's a separate disorder in which your kidneys eliminate too much fluid from your body.

SYMPTOMS OF DIABETES

diabetes symptoms are caused by increased blood sugar.

General symptoms
The general symptoms of diabetes include:
- increased hunger
- increased thirst
- weight loss
- frequent urination
- blurry eyesight
- terrible fatigue
- sores that don't heal.

Symptoms in men

In addition to the normal symptoms of diabetes, men with diabetes may have diminished sex desire, erectile dysfunction (ED), and inadequate physical strength.

Symptoms in women

Women with diabetes might also experience symptoms such as urinary tract infections, yeast infections, and dry, itchy skin.

Type 1 diabetes

Symptoms of type 1 diabetes may include:

- intense hunger
- increased thirst

- unintentional weight loss
- frequent urination
- blurry vision
- tiredness
- It may also result in mood swings.

Type 2 diabetes

Symptoms of type 2 diabetes may include:

- increased hunger
- increased thirst
- increased urination
- blurry vision
- tiredness

wounds that are sluggish to heal

It may also cause recurrent infections. This is because increased glucose levels make it harder for the body to mend.

Gestational diabetes

Most women with gestational diabetes don't exhibit any symptoms. The problem is commonly diagnosed through a regular blood sugar test or oral glucose tolerance test that is normally conducted between the 24th and 28th weeks of gestation.

In rare situations, a woman with gestational diabetes may also suffer increased thirst or urination.

Bottom line

Diabetes symptoms might be so faint that they're hard to recognize at first. Learn which indicators should trigger a trip to the doctor.

CAUSES OF DIABETES

Different reasons are connected with each type of diabetes.

Causes of type 1 diabetes

Doctors don't know precisely what causes type 1 diabetes. For whatever reason, the immune system erroneously assaults and kills insulin-producing beta cells in the pancreas.

Genes may have a role in certain persons. It's also conceivable that a virus kicks off the immune system onslaught.

Causes of type 2 diabetes

Type 2 diabetes originates from a mix of genetics and lifestyle factors. Being overweight or obese raises your risk too. Carrying excess weight, particularly in your belly, makes your cells more resistant to the effects of insulin on your blood sugar.

This disease runs in families. Family members share genes that make them more likely to have type 2 diabetes and to be overweight.

Causes of gestational diabetes

Gestational diabetes is the outcome of hormonal changes throughout pregnancy. The placenta generates hormones that make a pregnant woman's cells less susceptible to the effects of insulin. This may induce high blood sugar during pregnancy.

Women who are overweight when they are pregnant or who gain too much weight throughout their pregnancy are more likely to have gestational diabetes.

Bottom line

Both factors (genes and environmental factors) have a role in generating diabetes. Get more information on further chapters about the causes of diabetes.

DIABETES RISK FACTORS

Certain things raise your chance of diabetes.

Type 1 diabetes risk factors

You're more likely to have type 1 diabetes if you're a kid or adolescent, you have a parent or sibling with the illness, or you inherit particular genes that are connected to the disease.

Type 2 diabetes risk factors

Your risk for type 2 diabetes rises if you:

- are overweight
- are age 45 or older
- have a parent or sibling with the condition
- aren't physically active
- have had gestational diabetes
- have prediabetes

- have high blood pressure, high cholesterol, or high triglycerides
- have African American, Hispanic or Latino American, Alaska Native, Pacific Islander, American Indian, or Asian American heritage

Gestational diabetes risk factors

Your risk for gestational diabetes rises if you:

- are overweight
- are over age 25
- had gestational diabetes during a former pregnancy
- have given birth to a baby weighing more than 9 pounds
- have a family history of type 2 diabetes
- have polycystic ovary syndrome (PCOS) (PCOS)

The bottom line

Your family, environment, and prior medical issues may all impact your risks of having diabetes. Find out which hazards you can manage and which ones you can't.

DIABETES COMPLICATIONS

high blood sugar damages organs and tissues throughout your body. The higher your blood sugar is and the longer you live with diabetes, the greater your chance for problems.

Complications connected with diabetes include:

- heart illness, heart attack, and stroke
- neuropathy
- nephropathy
- retinopathy and vision loss
- hearing loss
- foot damage such as infections and sores that don't heal skin issues such as bacterial and fungal infections
- depression
- dementia

Gestational diabetes complications

Uncontrolled gestational diabetes may lead to issues that harm both the mother and baby. Complications impacting the infant might include:

- preterm births
- higher or overweight at birth increased risk for type 2 diabetes later in life
- slow blood sugar
- jaundice
- stillbirth
- The mother might develop issues like as high blood pressure (preeclampsia) or type 2 diabetes. She may also need cesarean delivery, generally referred to as a C-section.
- The mother's risk of gestational diabetes in future pregnancies also rises.

Diabetes can lead to serious medical complications, but you can manage the condition with medications and lifestyle changes. Avoid the most common diabetes complications with these helpful tips.

DIABETES DIAGNOSIS

Anyone who shows signs of diabetes or is at risk for the condition should be tested. Women are regularly screened for gestational diabetes throughout their second or third trimesters of pregnancy. Doctors use these blood tests to identify prediabetes and diabetes:

The fasting plasma glucose (FPG) test analyzes your blood sugar after you've fasted for 8 hours.

The A1C test offers a snapshot of your blood sugar levels over the last 3 months.

To diagnose gestational diabetes, your doctor will test your blood sugar levels between the 24th and 28th weeks of your pregnancy.

During the glucose challenge test, your blood sugar is measured one hour after you ingest a sweet beverage.

During the 3-hour glucose tolerance test, your blood sugar is measured after you fast overnight and then consume a sweet beverage.

The earlier you are diagnosed with diabetes, the sooner you can start treatment. Find out if you should be tested, and receive additional information about tests your doctor could do.

If you don't currently have a primary care specialist, you may research providers in your region for more online or media platforms.

DIABETES PREVENTION

Type 1 diabetes isn't prevented since it's caused by an issue with the immune system. Some causes of type 2 diabetes, such as your genes or age, aren't under your control either.

Yet many other diabetes risk factors are controlled. Most diabetes preventive options include making easy modifications to your diet and workout program.

If you've been diagnosed with prediabetes, here are a few things you can take to postpone or avoid type 2 diabetes:

Get at least 150 minutes each week of cardiovascular activity, such as walking or cycling.

Cut saturated and trans fats, along with processed carbs, out of your diet.

Eat more fruits, veggies, and healthy grains.

Eat lesser servings.

Try to drop 7 percent of the trusted Source of your body weight if you're overweight or obese.

These aren't the only approaches to avoiding diabetes. Discover additional measures that may help you prevent this chronic condition In further chapters of this book.

DIABETES IN PREGNANCY

Women who've never had diabetes might suddenly acquire gestational diabetes in pregnancy. Hormones generated by the placenta may make your body more resistant to the effects of insulin.

Some women who had diabetes before they conceived carry it with them into pregnancy. This is termed pre-gestational diabetes. Gestational diabetes should go away once you deliver, but it does considerably raise your chance of acquiring diabetes later.

About half of women with gestational diabetes may acquire type 2 diabetes within 5 to 10 years after birth, according to the International Diabetes Federation (IDF) (IDF).

Having diabetes during your pregnancy might potentially lead to difficulties for your infant, such as jaundice or breathing problems.

If you're diagnosed with pre-gestational or gestational diabetes, you'll require careful monitoring to avoid problems. Find out more about the effect of diabetes on pregnancy.

Diabetes in children

Children may have both type 1 and type 2 diabetes. Controlling blood sugar is particularly critical in young individuals, since the condition may harm key organs such as the heart and kidneys.

Type 1 diabetes in children.

The autoimmune type of diabetes generally develops in infancy. One of the primary signs is excessive urination. Kids with type 1 diabetes may start wetting the bed after they've been toilet trained.

Extreme thirst, weariness, and hunger are additional indications of the disease. It's vital that children with type 1 diabetes receive treatment straight soon. The condition may induce excessive blood sugar and dehydration, which can constitute medical issues.

Type 2 diabetes in children.

Type 1 diabetes used to be termed "juvenile diabetes" since type 2 was so infrequent in youngsters. Now that more children are overweight or obese, type 2 diabetes is becoming increasingly widespread in this age range.

About 40 percent of children with type 2 diabetes don't show symptoms, according to the Mayo Clinic. The condition is generally identified during a physical checkup.

Untreated type 2 diabetes may bring lifelong problems, including heart disease, renal disease, and blindness. Healthy nutrition and exercise may help your kid regulate their blood sugar and avoid these complications.

Type 2 diabetes is more widespread than ever in young individuals. Learn how to spot the signs so you can report them to your child's doctor.

PLEASE NOTE !!!

 diabetes — like type 1 — is caused by factors that are out of your control. Others – like type 2 — may be avoided with improved eating choices, more exercise, and weight reduction.

CHAPTER 2

GOOD & HEALTHY FOODS FOR DIABETES

Eating a balanced diet may have a major influence on treating type 2 diabetes or avoiding prediabetes from becoming type 2 diabetes. Making a shopping list of healthful foods is one method that might help individuals with diabetes remain on track.

Choosing healthful, delicious meals that match specific dietary needs may also help persons with type 2 diabetes manage their disease.

The American Diabetes Association recommends customers always check the nutrition information label of a product. It is the greatest approach to knowing how many carbohydrates and how many calories are in the dish.

VEGETABLES

Vegetables constitute the backbone of a healthy diet. They are good sources of vitamins, minerals, and fiber.

Fiber and complex carbs, found in many veggies, might help a person feel full. This in turn helps inhibit overeating, which may lead to undesired weight gain and issues with blood sugar.

Some veggies to add to the shopping list include :

- broccoli
- carrots
- greens
- peppers
- tomatoes
- potatoes
- corn
- green peas

BEANS AND LEGUMES

Beans, lentils, and other pulses are rich sources of nutritional fiber and protein.

The high fiber component of foods of the pulse family implies that the digestive system absorbs fewer carbs than it does from low fiber, high carbohydrate diets.

This makes these items an ideal carbohydrate option for those with diabetes. People may also use them instead of meat or cheese.

Below are some samples of what beans should pick up in a canned or dried form:

- black beans
- lentils
- white beans
- garbanzo beans
- kidney beans
- pinto beans

Also, pressure- or slow-cooking beans may assist enhance their digestibility.

FRUITS

Fruit may have high sugar content, however, the sugar in whole fruit does not contribute to free sugars. Therefore, those with diabetes should not avoid fruit.

The following fruits make a great complement to the diet of anybody who has type 2 diabetes, due to their low glycemic index (GI) and glycemic load:

- apples
- avocado
- blackberries
- cherries.
- grapefruit
- peaches
- pears
- plums
- strawberries

WHOLE GRAINS

Whole grains may be an effective strategy for persons with diabetes to regulate their blood glucose levels, as they frequently have a lower GI.

People should avoid bleached and processed carbs, such as white bread and spaghetti, and instead pick some of the following when ingesting grains:

whole wheat or legume pasta
whole-grain bread with at least 3 grams of fiber per slice

- quinoa
- wild rice
- 100% whole-grain or whole wheat flour
- cornmeal
- oatmeal
- millet
- amaranth
- barley

Whole grains will also keep a person feeling full for longer, and they might have more taste than processed carbs.

DAIRY

Dairy products include vital nutrients, including calcium and protein. Certain evidence shows that dairy has a favorable impact on insulin secretion in some patients with type 2 diabetes.

Some of the greatest possibilities to add to one's diet are:

Parmesan, ricotta, or cottage cheese
low fat or skimmed milk
low-fat Greek or plain yogurt.

Meat Proteins are vital for persons with diabetes.
Similarly to high fiber and high-fat diets, proteins are slow to digest and generate only minor elevations in blood sugar.

The following are some excellent sources of protein to pick from:

- skinless,
- boneless chicken breast or strips
- salmon, sardines, tuna, and other oily fish
- white fish fillets
- skinless turkey breast
- eggs

Plant-based proteins include beans and bean derivatives, such as:
- black beans
- kidney beans

- pinto beans
- baked or refried beans
- hummus
- falafel
- lentils
- peas
- edamame
- tempeh
- tofu

Dressings, dips, spices, and condiments
Plenty of flavorings and dressings might be excellent for people seeking to regulate their blood sugar.
The following are some nice alternatives that persons with diabetes may pick from:
- vinegar
- olive oil
- mustard
- any spice or herb
- any kind of extracts
- hot sauces
- salsa

To prepare a vinaigrette, whisk together equal volumes of olive oil and balsamic or another vinegar then add salt, pepper, mustard, and herbs to taste.

Remember to account for the carbs a dressing delivers.

Barbecue sauces, ketchup, and some salad dressings may also be high in fat, sugar, or both, thus it is vital to read the nutrition information label before purchasing any of these items.

DESSERT FOODS

people with type 2 diabetes may enjoy sweets, but they should exercise caution when selecting portion sizes and how frequently they consume them.

The following are some of the low calorie or low carbohydrate dessert alternatives that have less of an influence on blood sugar levels than conventional desserts:

- popsicles with no added sugar
- 100 percent fruit popsicles dessert incorporating sugar-free gelatin pudding or ice cream sweetened with

zero-calorie or low-calorie sweeteners, such as stevia and erythritol

- Fruit-based sweets — such as homemade fruit salad without added sugar, or mixed summer fruits — may be a pleasant and healthful way to cap a meal.

It is recommended, however, to account for the sugar in fruit while measuring carbs.

Sugar-free solutions for diabetes

A person with diabetes will need to monitor their sugar consumption. However, sugar-free meals may still influence a person's blood glucose.

"Sugar-free" denotes that a food item does not have added sugar, but the product itself might contain carbs, which affect blood glucose levels.

One example of this is a sugar alcohol. Manufacturers typically employ these reduced-calorie sweeteners in sugar-free chewing gum, sweets, ice cream, and fruit spreads. Examples include:

- xylitol
- erythritol
- sorbitol
- maltitol

These are kinds of carbohydrates that may boost blood glucose levels.

A person may desire to select sugar replacements. In most circumstances, one serving of sugar replacement will not influence blood glucose levels.

Common sugar replacements include:
- saccharin
- neotame
- aspartame
- sucralose
- stevia
- SNACKS

For cravings between meals, a person might try:

- handmade popcorn, but not ready-made or sweetened varieties nuts, but not sweetened ones
- carrot or celery sticks with hummus
- modest quantities of fresh fruit coupled with a protein or fat, such as an apple with almond butter

DRINKS.

Water is healthful for everyone, including persons with diabetes.

There are other possibilities, however, beverages such as milk and juice may contain significant quantities of carbs and will affect a person's blood sugar. It is consequently vital to account for these like one would for food.

Here are a few choices a person with diabetes may desire to consider:
- unsweetened ice or hot tea
- unsweetened coffee
- low fat or skimmed milk
- unsweetened plant-based milks
- sparkling water

FOODS TO RESTRICT OR AVOID

people with type 2 diabetes should limit or avoid similar foods that are bad for folks without the illness. They should also avoid the items that cause large blood sugar changes.

A person should avoid diets with high quantities of simple carbohydrates saturated and trans fats

sugar in the shape of sweets, ice cream, and cakes

More precisely, consumers should restrict their consumption of:

packaged and quick meals, such as *baked goods,

- candy, chips,
- and desserts
- white bread
- white pasta
- white rice
- sweet cereals
- sugary drinks
- processed meat.

- red meat

It is also important to avoid low-fat items that have substituted fat with sugar. Fat-free yogurt is a nice example.

People living with prediabetes or type 2 diabetes might try substituting certain meals for healthier equivalents. This may include selecting wholemeal rice, pasta, or bread or substituting white potatoes with sweet potatoes or yams.

Homemade cuisine is typically the best choice since it is easy to eliminate the added sugars that are included in many ready-made food products.

CHAPTER 3

UNDERSTANDING FOOD PACKAGING

Food packaging may be perplexing. Most food products require a nutrition data label, but many consumers have difficulties reading it or understanding what to look for. Here are some helpful ideas for a better comprehension of package labels and messages:

Read the nutrition data label: That a food promises to be lower in fat or decreased sugar does not guarantee it truly is. It is vital to search for and go through the nutrition data label on the container to understand what the item contains.

Look for particular nutrition facts: The information might be perplexing for many individuals. The most crucial information for those with diabetes to look for is the number of carbs per serving and how large a portion is.

Count carbohydrates: Dietary fiber is a kind of carbohydrate, therefore it may show under the column for total carbs. The body does not digest dietary fiber, therefore a person may remove it from the total carbs in the meal. This is a more precise approach to counting the carbohydratesTrusted Source.

Read the components list: The list of components goes from the greatest total content to the lowest. If sugar is at the top, it is the major element.

Look for hidden sources of sugar: Sugar can hide in foods under many different names, including corn syrup, fructose, and dextrose. Being aware of sugar's numerous identities might help a buyer make safer decisions.

Limit or avoid artificial sweeteners: Older researchTrusted Source suggests that artificial sweeteners can harm health and can encourage sweet cravings. However, not all scientists who trusted Source agree. Some popular artificial sweeteners include aspartame, sucralose, neotame, saccharin, and acesulfame potassium.

Sample grocery list

A shopping list will normally change from week to week, dependent on a person's requirements and desires. However, people may desire to explore the following example list to get started:

- Cucumber
- Apples
- tomatoes
- whole strawberries
- fresh or frozen vegetables or both
- Corn
- fresh basil
- a salad bag
- onion
- red bell pepper
- romaine lettuce
- yellow or green squash or zucchini boneless, skinless chicken breasts
- wild-caught salmon fillet
- unsweetened almond or flax milk
- 1–2% milk

- fresh mozzarella cheese
- Parmesan cheese
- sweet potatoes
- wild rice mix
- honey
- unsweetened, olive oil-based dressing
- low sugar, low sodium barbecue sauce
- olive oil
- olive oil spray
- black pepper
- reduced-sodium soy sauce
- salt
- coffee
- walnuts, almonds, or other raw nuts

impact of diet on diabetes

Several things may impact diabetes treatment. A person may handle several of them, including:

- what they consume,
- how much of it, and how often
- their carbohydrate intake

- how often do they measure their blood sugar
- the quantity of physical activity they engage in
- the accuracy and consistency of any medication doses they use
- sleep length and quality

Even slight changes in one of these areas might alter blood sugar regulation.

When a person eats thoughtfully, monitors meal quantities every day includes daily physical exercise, enjoy restful sleep, and takes medicine as instructed, they may improve their blood sugar levels dramatically.

With effective glucose control comes a decreased chance of consequences such as heart disease, coronary artery disease, renal disease, and nerve damage.

It is also crucial for individuals to regulate what they eat and boost physical exercise if suitable. This may help a person attain or maintain reasonable body weight.

FOODS FOR OTHER CONDITIONS

Diabetes may occur with other illnesses, such as renal and cardiovascular disease.

In certain circumstances, the nutritional demands for these distinct conditions alter relatively little. In other circumstances, a person may need to observe their diet considerably more strictly. Doing this may help address some of their symptoms.

A person may consult a doctor or nutritionist for dietary recommendations.

Below, we provide examples of foods to take or avoid with various coexisting conditions:

Diabetes and hypertension

People with high blood pressure, or hypertension, plus diabetes may follow a similar dietary regimen to those with simply diabetes.

However, those with hypertension should also restrict salt and caffeine consumption.

A person with both diabetes and hypertension should:

pick meals with reduced sodium levels

avoid or minimize coffee and caffeinated drinks

avoid or restrict meals that are rich in saturated and trans fats

Diabetes and celiac disease

People with celiac disease need to avoid goods containing wheat, barley, and rye since their systems are unable to digest the gluten that is contained in these products.

A person with both celiac disease and type 2 diabetes should examine food labels to verify the food they purchase is free from gluten.

Diabetes and obesity

People with obesity and diabetes should follow the same food rules as people with only diabetes.

For example, it is a good idea to:

Avoid or restrict foods rich in carbs and saturated and trans fats

monitor portion sizes, particularly in the case of meals that include carbs, fat, or both limit salt consumption to assist minimize the consequences from high blood pressure

The ideal approach is to adopt a balanced diet consisting of fruit, vegetables, lean proteins, and high-fiber carbs.

dietician or doctor can assist establish a meal plan that is suitable to each individual's requirements and lifestyle.

CHAPTER 4

JUNK FOOD AND DIABETES: TIPS FOR EATING OUT

Diabetes-friendly solutions

Diabetes is a disease when the body is unable to create enough insulin or utilize it appropriately. Diet is vital for treating diabetes and avoiding complications.

The body requires insulin to manage levels of sugar, or glucose, in the blood and to utilize this sugar to power the body's cells. Without insulin, the body cannot digest glucose, which comes from carbs in the diet. When excessive quantities of glucose gather in the blood, over time, they might harm the body's organs as the blood circulates. In addition, the body's cells would not have enough energy, since, without insulin, glucose cannot reach the cells.

Healthful eating is a key technique for regulating blood sugar levels. A person with a new diagnosis of diabetes may have to reassess their diet.

This might seem difficult, however, by making sensible choices, it is feasible for persons with diabetes to enjoy their favorite meals — even junk foods — from time to time and in moderation.

What is the link?

Junk food is heavy in calories and sugar but lacking in nutrition.

Junk foods are unhealthful foods. They are generally heavy in calories fat, sugar, salt, and processed carbs, and poor in beneficial nutrients, such as fiber, vitamins, and minerals.

Junk food encompasses numerous varieties of fast food, processed meals, and prepackaged snack items.

People should consume these items seldom, particularly if they have diabetes.

Possible consequences

Junk foods may contribute to diabetes in the following ways:

Rapid impact on blood sugar levels: Highly processed meals that are rich in calories and poor in vitamins, minerals, and fiber break down fast in the body and may produce a rapid spike in blood sugar levels.

Inappropriate portion size: Junk meals are typically not particularly filling and sometimes come in huge serving sizes. Both these variables may encourage individuals to consume junk foods. This may have a bad influence on diabetes, including blood sugar increases and weight gain.

Weight gain: Due to its low nutritional properties and potential to induce overeating, persons who consume junk food may gain weight. Excess weight and body fat are key risk factors for developing type 2 diabetes, which accounts for 90–95 percent of trusted sources of all instances of diabetes.

High blood pressure: Junk food is frequently particularly rich in sodium (salt), which leads to high blood pressure. High blood pressure is connected to an increased risk of type 2 diabetes.

Triglyceride levels: Junk foods are rich in trans and saturated fats, which may boost levels of triglycerides, a form of fat that is present in the blood. High levels of triglycerides raise the chance of acquiring type 2 diabetes.

According to a 2016 study trusted Source published in Experimental Physiology, habitually consuming junk foods may do as much harm to the kidneys of persons without diabetes as it does to those with the condition itself. Junk food also produces high blood sugar levels comparable to those seen by persons with type 2 diabetes.

As persons with diabetes are already at a greater risk of kidney damage, diets including a lot of junk foods may be extremely dangerous.

Saturated and trans fats

Nuts, seeds, avocado, and olive oil are all beneficial fats.

The American Diabetes Association suggests consuming fewer saturated and trans fats to minimize the risk of heart disease, which may be a consequence of diabetes.

Saturated fat elevates blood cholesterol levels and triglyceride levels. Health officials suggest that fewer than 10 percent of a person's daily calorie intake comes from saturated fats.

For a person on a 1,800-calorie diet, this implies they may ingest 20 grams of saturated fat in a day. This may be tough to perform on a diet involving junk foods.

Sources of saturated fat include:
- chicken and turkey skin
- chocolate
- dairy items (butter, cheese, cream, ice cream, whole milk, sour cream) (butter, cheese, cream, ice cream, whole milk, sour cream).
- ground beef

- hot dogs
- lard
- palm oilpork,
- comprising sausage,
- bacon, ribs, and fatback pork

A review paper published in 2016 revealed that trans fats might have a detrimental influence on insulin sensitivity and raise the incidence of type 2 diabetes, however, the study author emphasizes that additional research is essential.

Sources of trans fats include:
- crackers and chips
- cookies
- fast food items, including fries hydrogenated oil or partly hydrogenated oil margarines
- muffins and cakes
- shortening

When determining levels of trans fat in a product, note that food manufacturers may label their item as having 0 grams (g) of trans fats if the product contains less than 0.5 g.

In 2015, the Food and Drug Administration Trusted Sourcedetermined that partially hydrogenated oils, a primary source of trans fat, are not "Generally Recognized As Safe (GRAS)."

They have subsequently outlawed the introduction of partly hydrogenated oils to meals. All food firms have until January 1, 2020, to eliminate these oils from their present food production processes.

Carbs : Understanding both amount and type of carbohydrates are vital in treating diabetes. Balancing insulin levels in the body with carbohydrate consumption is crucial to maintaining blood glucose levels.

Heavily processed and junk meals generally include added sugar, a fast-acting carbohydrate that may rapidly elevate insulin levels.

They also tend to include process, rather than whole, grains and so lack the minerals and fiber that slows down the body's digestion of carbs.

The number and kinds of carbohydrates that a person with diabetes should take differs between people. It depends on a lot of parameters, including height, weight, exercise level, and the usage of drugs. A doctor or dietician will advise on a proper quantity for each individual.

<u>Tips</u>

It is crucial to read the nutritional information of store-bought food and comprehend per serving quantities.

Education and planning are crucial to making the best beneficial choices while dining out, particularly when picking junk food.

- Many restaurants, especially major chain restaurants, post the nutrition composition of their cuisine online.
- It is a good idea to check these websites before dining out or to obtain nutritional information at the restaurant.

- Learn how to interpret the nutritional information on store-bought convenience and snack items, paying special attention to total calories, carbs, fat, and salt levels.
- The list will display nutrition information per serving, so be careful to look at the serving size and understand quantities based on this.

Some strategies for better fast food choices

- Don't be scared to make specific demands. Ask servers to leave out particular goods, or exchange them for others.Request smaller servings and ask for sauces and dressings on the side, or do not have them at all. Consider ordering side salads to start instead of the main meal, or go for an appetizer with some nutritious sides.
- Avoid premium or super-sized meals at fast food establishments. These may

save money but are heavier in calories, fat, and sugar.

- Ask for dishes without full-fat dressings or sauces, such as mayonnaise, ranch, or other creamy sauces. Mustard or fat-free dressings are healthier alternatives. Ketchup commonly includes high fructose corn syrup, thus individuals should be aware of their use of this condiment since it might increase blood sugar.
- Choose a salad or veggie-based meal where possible, with grilled chicken, fish, tofu, or beans. Add a low-fat dressing on the side.
- Order burgers sans cheese. Ask for more salad toppings instead, if desired.
- Try an open-faced burger, with just half of a bun, or no bread. Or, go for a lettuce wrap.
- Choose sides carefully. Instead of french fries or potato chips, go for side salads, fresh fruit, or raw veggies.

- Pizzas are healthier if they feature whole-wheat thin crusts, vegetable toppings, mild cheese, or no cheese at all. One recommendation is to have a side salad before eating pizza, since this may assist reduce overeating.
- It is better to avoid fried or breaded fish or poultry and pick grilled or broiled varieties.
- When dining from salad bars, pick non-starchy veggies, such as leafy greens, carrots, bell peppers, broccoli, and cucumber. Nuts, seeds, and avocado are healthy fat alternatives. Avoid or restrict cheese, bacon, and mayonnaise-based foods.
- Sodas, smoothies, and fruit juices may provoke blood sugar rises. Plain or sparkling water or unsweetened tea are preferable alternatives.
- Restaurant servings tend to be large. Find out the principles concerning nutritious portion sizes and follow them. For example, 3 ounces of

cooked fowl or fish is the size of a deck of cards, 1 tablespoon of dressing is the size of an adult thumb, and a clenched fist amounts to around 1 cup.

- Use the "plate method" and fill half the plate with non-starchy vegetables, one quarter with lean meat, fish, tofu, or beans, and one quarter with healthy grains and starchy veggies. Add a piece of fruit and a cup of low-fat milk or water. Be cautious of how huge the platter is. These suggestions are for a 9-inch plate.

CHAPTER 5

RECOMMENDED EXERCISES FOR DIABETES

If you live with type 2 diabetes, exercising frequently may help you control your blood sugar levels and weight. It may also help you minimize your risk of heart attack and stroke, reduce cardiovascular risk factors, and boost general health and well-being. Exercise may also help prevent the development of diabetes in persons who have prediabetes. The American Diabetes Association (ADA) urges patients to acquire at least 150 minutes of moderate-intensity aerobic exercise each week.

The advantages of exercise are independent of weight reduction. However, compliance with a workout regimen needs to be constant in order to see permanent improvements.

If you're sedentary and contemplating beginning an exercise program, it's a good idea to visit a doctor first to make sure there are no limits or particular precautions. It's usually a good idea to start cautiously and work up to your particular objective.

Not sure where to start? Here are several workouts that might help you attain your fitness objectives.

1. Walking

You don't need a gym membership or pricey workout equipment to begin moving.

If you have a sturdy set of shoes and a secure area to walk, you may start now. In fact, you may reach your suggested minimum objective for aerobic fitness by going for a brisk 30-minute walk five days per week.

According to a 2021 review, walking may assist persons with type 2 diabetes to decrease their blood pressure, HbA1c levels, and body mass index.

2. Cycling

Roughly half of the patients with type 2 diabetesTrusted Source have arthritis. The two illnesses have various risk factors in common, including obesity.

Diabetic neuropathy, a disorder that arises when the nerves get destroyed, may also cause joint discomfort in persons with type 2 diabetes.

If you have lower joint discomfort, try adopting low-impact activity. Cycling, for example, may help you reach your fitness objectives while avoiding pressure on your joints.

3. Swimming

Aquatic activities are another joint-friendly workout alternative. For example, swimming, water aerobics, aqua jogging, and other aquatic exercises may offer your heart, lungs, and muscles a workout, while placing minimal stress on your joints.

A 2017 review revealed that water exercise may assist reduce blood sugar levels, just like land-based exercise does.

4. Team sports

If you find it hard to encourage yourself to exercise, it could help to join a leisure sports team. The chance to mingle with colleagues and the commitment you make to them could help you discover the drive you need to show up each week.

Many leisure activities give a strong cardio exercise. Consider attempting basketball, soccer, softball, couples tennis, or ultimate frisbee.

5 . Aerobic dance

Signing up for aerobic dancing or other fitness programs could also help you accomplish your activity objectives. For instance, Zumba is a fitness program that blends dance and aerobic motions for fast-paced exercise.

A 2015 study discovered that women with type 2 diabetes were more motivated to exercise after taking part in Zumba lessons for 16 weeks. Participants also increased their aerobic fitness and dropped weight.

6. Weightlifting

Weightlifting and other strengthening exercises help improve your muscle mass, which may boost the number of calories you burn each day. Strength exercise may also assist improve your blood sugar management, according to the ADA.

If you want to add weightlifting to your weekly training program, you may use weight machines, free weights, or even heavy household items, such as canned goods or water bottles.

To learn how to lift weights safely and successfully, try taking a weightlifting class or contacting a professional fitness trainer for advice.

7. Resistance band workouts

Weights aren't the only instrument you may employ to improve your muscles. You may also undertake a broad range of strengthening exercises using resistance bands.

To understand how to integrate them into your exercises, chat with a professional trainer, attend a resistance band class, or watch a resistance band training video.

In addition to enhancing your strength, exercising with resistance bands may bring small improvements to your blood sugar management, according to 2018 research.

8. Calisthenics

In calisthenics, you use your own body weight to build your muscles. Common calisthenic workouts include pushups, pullups, squats, lunges, and belly crunches.

Whether you want to develop your muscles using weights, resistance bands, or your own body weight, aim to work out every major muscle group in your body.

To allow your body time to heal, experts advocate taking a day off from muscle-strengthening exercises between each session of strength training.

9. Pilates

Pilates is a popular fitness program that's designed to improve core strength, coordination, and balance. According to a 2020 study of older adult women with type

2 diabetes, it may also help improve blood sugar control.

Consider signing up for a Pilates class at your local gym or Pilates studio. Many instructive videos and books are also available.

10. Yoga

According to a 2016 analysis, yoga may assist persons with type 2 diabetes control their blood sugar, cholesterol levels, and weight. It could also help decrease your blood pressure, enhance the quality of your sleep, and raise your mood.

If you're interested in attempting yoga, sign up for a session at a local studio or gym. A skilled practitioner can assist you to learn how to transition from one position to another, utilizing the right posturc and breathing technique.

Exercise safety

Always consult with your doctor before beginning a new workout plan. In general, ensuring you're well hydrated before, during, and after activity.

Be sure to closely check your blood sugar levels as well to maintain them within your goal range.

CHAPTER 6

REVERSING TYPE 2 DIABETES & OBESITY

Type 2 Diabetes is a condition that is distinguished by persistently increased blood sugar levels. However, the major reason, as well as the driver for this illness, is something called Insulin Resistance. When you ingest certain meals, especially refined carbs, that food gets turned into sugar within your body. Your body's approach to coping with this sugar is to release a hormone called insulin. Insulin transfers the sugar within your cells so that it may be utilized for energy. Sounds amazing, right?

Well, yes and no. When operating properly, this is a terrific mechanism that assists your body to perform smoothly. But when you have type 2 diabetes, prediabetes, or considerable abdominal obesity, that mechanism does not perform so effectively.

Eating too many refined carbs boosts your insulin levels for lengthy periods of time and your cells start to develop resistance to the effects of insulin. Think of this a little like booze. When you start to drink, a single glass of wine might make you feel inebriated. Once your body grows habituated to drinking, you need more and more alcohol to produce the same impact. This is what occurs with diabetes. You need more and more insulin to perform the same thing. The difficulty is that too much insulin is poisonous to the body.

It is absolutely crucial to state that I do not think that there is one optimal diet for everyone. Different individuals react to different diets.

However, if you have a diagnosis of type 2 diabetes or if you have been informed you are at high risk or if you have considerable abdominal obesity, here are strategies to start reversing the effects immediately:

** **Avoid ALL refined carbs.*** That means no pasta, rice, or bread (even wholegrain bread can increase your insulin)\s* Avoid ALL additional sugar. If your body is already in a position where you cannot metabolize carbs and sugars effectively, you are going to have to take efforts to entirely remove all sweets, at least in the short term.

** **Avoid ALL sweet beverages***. It is recommended to stick to water, tea, and coffee.

** **Do not be terrified of excellent quality, nutritious, natural fat*** – avocados, olives, almonds, etc. Don't worry about this causing you to put on weight. Research released in 2003 found that participants who supplemented their diet with almonds lost more weight than those who supplemented with so-called "healthy, complex carbs"

** **Do not spend your efforts calculating calories***. Concentrate on the quality of the food that you are consuming and the calorie restriction will take care of itself.

***FEED YOUR GUT BUGS, not just yourself.** There are millions of microorganisms that dwell in your gut — their health is crucial in deciding your health. Many studies show correlations between the status of your gut bugs (your microbiota) and type 2 diabetes. Start boosting the health of your stomach immediately by eating five servings of various colored veggies each day. The nondigestible fiber in veggies is the preferred diet for your gut bacteria and when your gut bugs are happy, you will be pleased. The bigger the diversity of hues, the more phytonutrients you will be obtaining.

***If you want to nibble, carry some high-fat healthy snacks with you, such as olives, almonds, or hummus**. When you nibble on refined carbs such as biscuits, you go on a blood sugar rollercoaster that results in you feeling hungry immediately after. Fats, on the other hand, will keep you fuller for longer.

*** Include high-quality protein and fat with EVERY single meal.** This helps to balance your blood glucose and promotes satiety and fullness, making it less likely that you will want to go for dessert after your meal.

*** Eat your meals sitting down at a table.** Eating on the couch while watching TV fosters a thoughtless kind of eating — this might cause you to consume bigger amounts than you normally would. If you sit at a table and focus on what you're eating, you are more likely to enjoy your food, feel content at the conclusion of your meal, and eat less.

*** Consider a kind of regular fastings such as intermittent fasting or time-restricted eating (TRF) (TRF).** TRF involves consuming your calories within a certain window of the day and opting not to consume food for the remainder. It's a terrific technique to lower insulin levels in your body and help erase the consequences of persistently increased levels.

CHAPTER 7

LIFESTYLE CHANGES TO HELP MANAGE DIABETES

Working together with your doctor, you may control your diabetes by concentrating on these few important improvements in your everyday life.

1. Eat healthily. This is vital when you have diabetes, since what you consume impacts your blood sugar. No foods are off-limits. Focus on eating just as much as your body requires. Get lots of veggies, fruits, and healthy grains. Choose nonfat dairy and lean meats. Limit foods that are heavy in sugar and fat. Remember that carbs convert into sugar, so manage your carb consumption. Try to keep it around the same from meal to meal. This is much more crucial if you use insulin or medicines to regulate your blood sugars.

2. Exercise. If you're not active now, it's time to start. You don't have to join a gym and perform cross-training. Just walk, ride a bike, or play active video games. Your objective should be 30 minutes of action that makes you sweat and breathe a bit harder most days of the week. An active lifestyle helps you regulate your diabetes by bringing down your blood sugar. It also decreases your risk of having heart disease. Plus, it might help you reduce excess pounds and alleviate tension.

3. Get checks. See your doctor at least twice a year. Diabetes enhances your risk of heart disease. So memorize your numbers: cholesterol, blood pressure, and A1c (average blood sugar over 3 months) (average blood sugar over 3 months). Get a comprehensive eye checkup every year. Visit a foot doctor to check for concerns including foot ulcers and nerve damage.

4. Manage stress. When you're anxious, your blood sugar levels go up. And when you're nervous, you may not control your diabetes properly. You may forget to exercise, eat well, or take your prescriptions.

Find methods to release stress — through deep breathing, yoga, or activities that soothe you.

5. Stop smoking. Diabetes makes you more likely to have health issues such as heart disease, eye disease, stroke, kidney disease, blood vessel disease, nerve damage, and foot difficulties. If you smoke, your probability of acquiring these issues is significantly greater. Smoking also might make it tougher to exercise. Talk with your doctor about strategies to stop.

6. Watch your alcohol. It may be simpler to regulate your blood sugar if you don't get too much beer, wine, and liquor. So if you want to drink, don't overdo it. The American Diabetes Association states that women who consume alcohol should have no more than one drink a day and males should have no more than two. Alcohol might cause your blood sugar to go too high or too low. Check your blood sugar before you drink, and take efforts to prevent low blood sugars. If you use insulin or take medicines for your diabetes, eat while you're drinking.

OVERALL REMINDERS

<u>WHAT YOU SHOULDN'T DO WHEN DIABETIC:</u>

Patients who are on insulin or oral hypoglycemic agents should not fast, since it may result in hypoglycemia (low blood sugar levels).

They should not miss a meal expecting that it can be made up by eating additional food at the next meal. This may result in low blood sugar and also blood glucose swings which leads to microvascular problems.

- Do not consume white bread, chips, and pastries, which rapidly raise blood sugar.
- Avoid processed meals and meats since they will be heavy in salt and oil.
- Restrict fried and fatty meals.
- Do not consume full-fat dairy products.
- Alcohol raises blood pressure and triglycerides and excessive drinking damages the heart

- muscle (cardiomyopathy) (cardiomyopathy). In excess, it damages the liver and peripheral nerves.
- Do not use artificial sweeteners beyond the prescribed amount. If possible get accustomed to tea/coffee without sugar gradually.
- Do not work out on empty or full stomach.
- Do not watch TV when eating meals.
- Do not smoke.
- Do not miss your medicine.